# NHS: What's wrong and how to put it right

**Vernon Coleman**

# The author

Sunday Times bestselling author Vernon Coleman qualified as a doctor in 1970 and has worked both in hospitals and as a principal in general practice. Since 1975, he has written over 100 books which have sold over two million copies in the UK, been translated into 26 languages and sold all over the world. Several of his books have been on the bestseller lists. (There is a list of his books at the back of this book.) He has written over 5,000 articles in national newspapers and magazines and has presented numerous programmes on television and radio. His novel 'Mrs Caldicot's Cabbage War' was turned into a popular and award winning movie. Since 1999 he has been very happily married to the artist Donna Antoinette Coleman, with whom he has co-written five books. They live in the delightful if isolated village of Bilbury in Devon where they have designed for themselves a unique world to sustain and nourish them in these dark and difficult times.

# Vernon Coleman: What the papers say

'Vernon Coleman writes brilliant books.' – The Good Book Guide
'No thinking person can ignore him.' – The Ecologist
'The calmest voice of reason.' – The Observer
'A godsend.' – Daily Telegraph
'Superstar.' – Independent on Sunday
'Brilliant!' – The People
'Compulsive reading.' – The Guardian
'His message is important.' – The Economist
'He's the Lone Ranger, Robin Hood and the Equalizer rolled into one.' – Glasgow Evening Times
'The man is a national treasure.' – What Doctors Don't Tell You
'His advice is optimistic and enthusiastic.' – British Medical Journal
'Revered guru of medicine.' – Nursing Times
'Gentle, kind and caring' – Western Daily Press
'His trademark is that he doesn't mince words. Far funnier than the usual tone of soupy piety you get from his colleagues.' – The Guardian
'Dr Coleman is one of our most enlightened, trenchant and sensitive dispensers of medical advice.' – The Observer
'I would much rather spend an evening in his company than be trapped for five minutes in a radio commentary box with Mr Geoffrey Boycott.' – Peter Tinniswood, Punch
'Hard hitting...inimitably forthright.' – Hull Daily Mail
'Refreshingly forthright.' – Liverpool Daily Post
'Outspoken and alert.' – Sunday Express
'Dr Coleman made me think again.' – BBC World Service
'Marvellously succinct, refreshingly sensible.' – The Spectator
'Probably one of the most brilliant men alive today.' – Irish Times
'King of the media docs.' – The Independent
'Britain's leading medical author.' – The Star
'Britain's leading health care campaigner.' – The Sun
'Perhaps the best known health writer for the general public in the world today.' – The Therapist
'The patient's champion.' – Birmingham Post

'A persuasive writer whose arguments, based on research and experience, are sound.' – Nursing Standard
'The doctor who dares to speak his mind.' – Oxford Mail
'He writes lucidly and wittily.' – Good Housekeeping

Copyright Vernon Coleman August 2022
The right of Vernon Coleman to be identified as the author of this work has been asserted in accordance with the Copyright, Designs and Patents Act 1988.

To Antoinette
With all my love, always and all ways

**Contents**
Part One: What went wrong with the NHS and why
Part Two: How to mend the broken NHS
Part Three: A Better Alternative

# Part One
## What went wrong with the NHS – and why

It is easy to show that health care in Britain is worse today than it was 50 years ago. And arguably it is worse than it was 70 years ago. Indeed, it is worse than would be acceptable in many backward, third-world countries.

Health care in Britain has been doing more harm than good for many years because the NHS, which provides most of the health care in the UK, is dangerous, absurdly bureaucratic and wildly expensive. It has been dying for a long time.

I doubt if I was the only person to be shocked when the queen of England gave the George Cross medal to the NHS. The medal was apparently awarded to celebrate the way the NHS dealt with patients in 2020 and 2021. Those were the years when hospital departments were closed, for no good reason, when staff panicked and behaved hysterically in the face of an infection proven to be no more dangerous than the annual flu, when essential treatments were abandoned and waiting lists allowed to grow to inhuman proportions – with the result that millions of patients will die because they have not been investigated or treated. They were years when doctors and nurses wore masks which do more harm than good, and forced patients to wear them too. They were years when doctors and nurses ill-treated patients and were responsible for murdering tens, if not hundreds, of thousands of elderly patients simply because they were old and ill. They were years when doctors and nurses promoted, gave and lied about experimental, toxic jabs which never did what they were supposed to do but which were known to be among the most dangerous drugs ever manufactured. Worse still, doctors and nurses ignored the legal and ethical requirement to tell patients about all potential side effects before involving them in an experiment. They were years when doctors and nurses helped smear the honest practitioners who were trying to share the truth. They were the years when doctors and nurses mis-treated patients and betrayed every tenet of the Hippocratic Oath.

And it was because of all those sins that the queen gave the NHS staff the George Cross.

Of course, the queen has never had to use the NHS. The British taxpayers pay for her and her grasping, hypocritical, entitlement obsessed family to have the very best private care. It isn't because they live healthy lives or come from good genetic stock that most of them live such long lives. Their longevity is down to the fact that they receive private medical care and are not exposed to the inadequacies of the National Health Service.

You don't have to look far to find horror stories of maltreatment, neglect and incompetence. As I write, in August 2022, there are around seven million people waiting for urgent medical treatment and the figure is expected to double in the next twelve months. Millions more are waiting for essential tests to see if they have cancer or heart disease. And once the tests are done they will have to wait weeks or months for the results. There is effectively no GP service today. The average GP works just 26 hours a week and earns well over £100,000 (plus bonuses of between £50,000 and £100,000 for having their NHS nurse give covid jabs on their behalf). Many GPs refuse to see patients in the consulting room – and agree to telephone or video consultations only after patients have been interrogated by untrained reception staff. The vast majority of GPs refuse to visit patients at home (because the medical establishment decrees it a waste of their valuable time) and are not available even for telephone consultations outside their 26 hour working week. GPs are no longer available for evening or weekend calls and their surgeries are firmly shut at lunchtimes and on bank holidays. The result of the collapse of the GP service is that accident and emergency departments are clogged with patients usually having to wait eight or nine hours, and sometimes twice as long, to be seen in many hospitals. The queues for treatment are so long that ambulances (which now often take hours to respond to urgent, emergency calls for help) have to queue outside for up to 27 hours.

None of this has happened by accident.

The NHS was murdered and is clearly no longer fit for purpose; it is, on the face of it, an example to the world of the pointlessness and intrinsic design weakness of socialised medicine.

Although it might have been a tolerably good idea in 1948, years of reorganisation steadily gave the bureaucrats increasing authority, while at the same time diminishing the position of patients in the organisation and making the whole project vulnerable to the wishes of the conspirators who are now determined to push us into their Great Reset.

The NHS functioned reasonably well in the 1950s and 1960s, and even in the early 1970s but by the early 1980s the organisation was lost; taken over entirely by overpaid armies of men and women who had no knowledge of the principles of medical care and who believed that hospitals and clinics would run far more smoothly if patients were excluded. Administrators, like cockroaches, have no discernible value, multiply inexorably and are nigh on impossible to eradicate.

Over the last few decades the number of beds and nurses has gone down rapidly, just as the number of bureaucrats has risen. Today the NHS's more than ample funds are wasted on whole regiments of vastly overpaid bean counters and pen pushers. Patients have become an unnecessary burden; interfering in the smooth running of a large machine which is now designed solely and exclusively for the benefit of the parasitic hordes. And that is all deliberate. Doctors and nurses have lost heart. Nurses have become too important to nurse and lazy doctors, led by a ruinously powerful trade union, have become obsessed with status and money. The result is that the NHS provides a service that would not be tolerated in an old-fashioned Third World dictatorship. It is not surprising that most NHS staff now admit that they would not like to be treated in the hospital where they work and would not recommend the institution to friends or relatives. It is not surprising that most higher paid NHS staff now demand, and receive, private medical care cover for themselves and their families.

Things started to go wrong with the NHS half a century ago when appointment systems became more or less compulsory for GPs. Before that, patients had been able to see their family doctor simply by turning up at his or her surgery during the advertised opening hours. Patients who weren't well enough to visit the surgery, or weren't able to get there for any reason, could telephone for a home visit. And, of course, patients could telephone their doctor at any time of day or night, every day of the year, if they were ill or needed advice. The system worked well. Patients enjoyed the comfort of knowing that their doctor was pretty well instantly available, and doctors enjoyed the professional satisfaction of providing a personal, effective service to the patients on their list.

The introduction of appointment systems changed everything: turning GPs' surgeries into an administrative nightmare and providing new hurdles for patients to leap if they wanted advice. GPs who had managed with just a surgery, a waiting room, an office and one receptionist found that they needed extra staff to deal with the phone calls. Doctors who had run their practice from their homes, often using their dining room as a waiting room, had to move into purpose built health centres and clinics and hire extra receptionists to handle all the telephone calls and to keep the appointments book. Doctors found that they had to join together with other local practices because of the cost of the new clinics and the extra staff. The bureaucrats encouraged the development of clinics because they helped get rid of the traditional, lone GPs who had been difficult to control. As the clinics grew in size so the number of staff grew too. The dramatic increase in the number of receptionists meant that practice managers and personnel specialists had to be hired. When I first practised as a GP I managed with one member of staff – a receptionist. Today, my former practice has been submerged into an administrative giant – with dozens of employees.

As practices grew in size so doctors moved further and further away from their traditional roles.

In the old days, doctors used to do pretty well everything themselves. They took blood pressures, they weighed patients, they syringed ears, they took blood samples and so on. All these minor procedures helped to seal the relationship between doctors and patients. And because doctors regularly visited their patients in their homes, they grew to know them as people and, in many cases, as friends. The chronic sick knew to whom they could turn if they were worried about a hospital appointment or if they wanted a consultant's advice interpreted. The GP was the patient's valued first port of call in any illness, and remained the patient's advisor throughout any illness.

All that changed as practices grew in size. Doctors became remote figures; hiding behind teams of advisors and sub-specialists. When new employment laws from the European Union were brought in, it was decreed that GPs should not provide a 24 hour service for 365 days a year (even though very few GPs had complained about the system and, as far as I know, no patients had ever expressed dissatisfaction).When GPs were offered a chance to work the same sort of hours as librarians and accountants, their union leaders leapt at the opportunity and GPs abandoned their long-standing professional sense of responsibility. A system which demanded that there be more female doctors than male doctors suited the changes because female doctors wanted fewer working hours and no weekend or night work. They also found that by controlling their income they could dramatically reduce their tax liabilities. New laws were also introduced removing the traditional confidentiality which had always existed between doctors and patients and which had provided the bedrock for the sense of trust between the two. And GPs, now working part time at their NHS jobs, took on work for internet health companies. Patients who were unable to consult their own doctor found that they could, for a fee, consult a GP from another practice somewhere else in the country. GPs had created a demand for this new service by their own selfishness and greed.

And then nurses were encouraged to reconsider their position too.

From America, came the idea that nursing should be an academic rather than a practical profession. Leaders of the nursing profession demanded that nurses should be allowed to make diagnoses and to prescribe treatments. Only those nurses who took degrees and acquired academic certification were allowed to rise through the ranks to become senior members of the profession.

Before the 1970s, hospitals had been simply run. Each ward had a ward sister (who was in charge of the nursing) and a ward clerk (who was in charge of looking after the medical records). Each hospital had a matron (who was in charge of all nursing matters), a secretary (who was in charge of administration) and an almoner (who looked after patients' social problems). Porters were hired to wheel patients around and to look after the heavy work. Nursing auxiliaries dealt with simpler, routine nursing work.

All this worked well, to the quiet satisfaction of patients and staff, but it was changed dramatically by the introduction of many layers of administration.

The new administrators demanded more control and closed smaller hospitals because they did not fit comfortably into a new bureaucratic hierarchy which had been designed more for the satisfaction of the administrators than the welfare of patients or the comfort of the staff. Nurses and doctors abandoned working practices which had been carefully devised and perfected over generations and replaced them with selfish demands for greed and power.

In both general practice and hospitals, the bureaucrats had taken control. Aided and abetted by increasingly powerful professional trade unions which abandoned any sense of responsibility for patient care in favour of merely improving their members' earnings, the conspirators had successfully destroyed the National Health Service, removing all sense of morality from a system which had also become increasingly beholden to the powerful and corrupt international pharmaceutical industry.

What none of the unions realised, however, was that they had helped set up a system which was perfectly designed to ensure that individual professionals will, in just a few years, be completely replaced by robots and computers.

It has been proven time and time again that computers make better diagnosticians than doctors, that robots are better at surgery than human surgeons and that robots make better, more caring and more reliable nurses than human nurses. The robot nurses can be programmed with enough caring to revive the valuable placebo response that used to augment medical treatment in such a powerful way.

The health care trade unions haven't realised it yet but there is no future for human doctors or for human nurses. They will all be replaced by robots and computers. The new system, which eradicated home visits and destroyed the traditional relationship between doctors and patients, has made this possible.

The NHS could be rescued, if there was sufficient political will and if the medical and nursing professions could be persuaded or coerced into putting the interests of patients a little higher on their list of priorities.

But at the moment it is very easy to argue that the NHS today provides a far inferior service to the NHS of 1970. And it is not difficult to argue that the NHS today provides a far inferior service to the NHS of 1950.

# Part Two
## How to mend the broken NHS

Here is how the NHS could be restored to something of its former glory.

First, the much hated appointment systems used by GPs should be abandoned completely. GPs should be required to open their surgeries twice a day (morning and evening) and to invite any patient requiring treatment or advice to turn up without any appointment. Abandoning appointment systems will mean that GPs can fire 90% of their administrative staff. The savings for the NHS will be vast. There will be far less paperwork to do and GPs will have much more time for diagnosing and treating patients.

Second, GPs must be made to go back to offering a service for 24 hours a day on 365 days a year. It is not an arduous responsibility. GPs can form themselves into small groups of three or four doctors and share the night and weekend calls. The idea that sitting waiting for a possible call-out must count as 'work' is a nonsense which originated with the European Union and was doubtless designed to destroy health services as well as economies throughout the region. For decades, thousands of GPs managed to provide a 24 hour service without any great harm being done to their physical or mental health. Many GPs provided the service without partners or assistants, merely hiring a locum once a year for two weeks or so if they wanted to take a holiday. Doctors would no doubt find that they enjoyed their work considerably more if they offered a better and more comprehensive service.

Third, hospital consultants must choose between working for the NHS or working as private consultants, outside the NHS. At the moment, consultants are allowed to mix and match and this has been disastrous. Many surgeons, for example, work 9/11ths of their time for the NHS and forgo a small portion of their salary. In the rest of their working week they perform operations privately. It beggars belief that someone in government allowed this absurd system to be approved. One problem is that it is difficult to be sure consultants are giving the NHS the time it has paid for. The other problem is that consultants deliberately build up their NHS waiting lists in order to encourage patients to go privately – and then pay thousands of pounds for an operation which the NHS should provide free of charge. When I was a junior doctor, one consultant for whom I was working took a month's holiday and the registrar and I, by dint of working hard, succeeded in seeing all the patients on his waiting list. By the time the consultant returned to work there was no waiting list. He was furious. 'Why should anyone pay to see me privately?' he demanded. 'If there is no waiting list for NHS patients.'

Fourth, GPs must work full time within the NHS or choose to work privately all the time. The nonsensical system currently in operation allows GPs to enjoy all the security of the NHS while moonlighting for private companies (particularly internet health companies offering online diagnoses). This must stop. GPs who choose to accept the comfort and high pay of an NHS job must agree not to work for anyone else.

Fifth, GPs must stop doing consultations by video or zoom. It has been proved beyond doubt that it is impossible for doctors to provide a good, reliable service this way. Patients need to be seen live, in a consulting room or at home. Any doctor who fails to see patients in their consulting room should be fired.

Sixth, nine out of ten hospital administrators should be fired immediately – including all those earning over £100,000 a year. The savings to the NHS will be vast – particularly since these expensive bureaucrats all enjoy absurdly generous pensions and require expensively furnished offices, teams of assistants and secretaries and lavish expense accounts.

Seventh, drug companies should be banned from subsidising conferences or paying GPs or hospital doctors fees for giving lectures or writing articles for medical magazines. At the moment most post graduate education is subsidised by drug companies and it is not surprising, therefore, that the drug companies control who will speak and who will be allowed to educate doctors and nurses. At the moment any doctor deemed unacceptable to the drug companies will be banned. (I have personal experience of this absurd form of censorship.) For five decades I have been fighting the absurd myth that drug companies and doctors have prolonged life expectancy. This, I'm afraid, is a self-serving piece of propaganda which exists solely to promote the pharmaceutical industry and the medical profession. The simple fact is that at the end of the 19th century, and the beginning of the 20th century, infant mortality was horrendously high and the fact that babies often died before they reached their first birthday gave the impression that life expectancy for adults was lower than it was. If one baby dies just after birth, and another baby lives to be 80 then the average life expectancy is around 40 years. Better drinking water, better sewage facilities, better housing and better food mean that today it is uncommon for babies to die and as a result the infant mortality rate has improved dramatically. This, in turn, has had a dramatic effect on average life expectancy. If one baby in 100 dies just after birth, and the other 99 live to be 80 then the average life expectancy is close to 80 years. This statistical anomaly enables drug companies, and the medical establishment, to claim that they are responsible for improving life expectancy. In truth, very few major improvements have been made by medical science. The biggest development was the serendipitous discovery of antibiotics nearly a century ago. And the advantage antibiotics gave us over infections has been squandered by absurd overprescribing and by allowing farmers to give antibiotics to most or all of their cattle. These disastrous errors have led to the development of antibiotic resistant bacteria. Drug companies and doctors have had virtually no impact on life expectation. Indeed, it is possible to argue that, on balance, they have done more harm than good. Certainly, thirty years ago I produced clear evidence that doctors are one of the three biggest killers – alongside cancer and circulatory disease. But the medical establishment (and journalists bought by the pharmaceutical industry) continue with their favourite and most powerful lie, suggesting that they and they alone are responsible for improving life expectation. Naturally, they refuse to debate the myth because they know they will lose the debate.

Eighth, drug companies should also be banned from advertising their drugs – particularly in medical journals. Officially independent medical journals receive millions of pounds in drug company advertising and, it seems to me, that this must affect their true independence and their willingness to criticise the drug industry. Indeed, medical journals rarely if ever do criticise drug companies. In my 20s I was editor of a widely circulated medical journal which frequently ran articles criticising drug companies. On one occasion I was with the publisher when a drug company boss told him that they would only consider buying advertising space in the journal if I were sacked. A few weeks later I was fired. I believe it is the unwholesome connection between medical journals and drug companies which explains why drug companies are allowed to suppress research results which would, if published, be inconvenient. The huge expenditure on advertising also helps control the mainstream media.

Ninth, medical charities must lose their links with drug companies. At the moment many large charities are more or less controlled by drug companies. This is dangerous and leads to patients being given biased information – biased in the favour of specific drug companies selling products which may or may not be of value. I am also convinced that drug companies use charities to help suppress products and treatment methods which might prove commercially disadvantageous to them. I believe that it is drug companies which have helped create the myth that 'dementia' is synonymous with Alzheimer's Disease. In my book 'Dementia Myth', I point out that the words 'Alzheimer's' and 'dementia' are often thought to be the same thing and the result is chronic illness and huge profits for drug companies. The truth, however, is that most cases of dementia are curable if properly diagnosed.

Tenth, every Government committee and quango dealing with drugs has close links to the pharmaceutical industry. The links between drug companies and the Government are unacceptably close and need to be ended. Many of the official NHS and Government advisory bodies should be closed down because of their relationships with the industry, and those which remain should have no links with drug companies whatsoever. The MHRA, for example, was given a donation of £980,000 for 'collaborating' with the Bill and Melinda Gates Foundation.

Eleventh, the Government must stop making payments to doctors and hospitals for making specific diagnoses. For example, the number of patients diagnosed with Alzheimer's Disease has been falsely enhanced by the fact that GPs receive an extra fee every time they diagnose the disease. Hospital policies have been distorted by the fact that hospitals are paid a bonus every time they diagnose covid-19.

Twelfth, doctors should not receive an extra fee every time they give a vaccination. The extra fees can add up to a huge amount of money (I have estimated that many doctors made £50,000 to £100,000 each from giving the covid jab.) If doctors simply gave vaccinations which they knew to be useful and safe there would be far less vaccinating going on. It is difficult to see why doctors should receive an extra bonus payment simply for doing their jobs. It is as absurd as paying Marks and Spencer staff a bonus every time they sell a pair of socks or a croissant. The whole vaccination programme needs properly assessing (something which has never been done, since new vaccinations are simply added to the collection without any testing to see how safe or effective these additions might be.) One of the many unfortunate side effects of the attention which has been given to the covid-19 jabs is the fact that more traditional vaccinations (including the dozens routinely given to children) have been forgotten and are now largely administered without protest, controversy or a second thought. Independent doctors need to assess the ever-growing hailstorm of vaccinations, aimed particularly at children, which have seemingly become an integral part of our relationship with health care in general and doctors in particular. There has for a long time been a blackout on any discussion of the more traditional vaccines and the reputation of vaccines is built on a toxic mixture of myths, fallacies and plain, vanilla lies. My own questioning of official establishment policies had, for a long time, made me unpopular with the establishment. Vaccination is a taboo subject and vaccines are protected from criticism in the way that film stars were protected in the 1930s. In 2011, I described vaccination as 'a massive confidence trick' and predicted that 'vaccination will become compulsory'. However, the mainstream media has devoted itself to promoting vaccines and never allowing any aspect of vaccination to be questioned. The BBC actually has a policy of excluding all vaccine criticism from its programmes. Merely questioning the validity of vaccination draws a torrent of abuse down upon the questioner's head. The inevitable result is that vaccination programmes continue pretty well unhindered and millions of children are now regularly jabbed with products which have never been properly tested or evaluated either for safety or efficacy. All around the world, infants and children are now subjected to a seemingly endless series of assaults on their immune systems. The vaccines used have never been adequately tested to see how they might interact or how they might affect other medications. Very few long-term trials have been done though the few available confirm my scepticism. For example, in 2017, the Danish Government and a Danish vaccine maker funded a study of the DTP vaccine. The WHO and the medical establishment claim that the DTP vaccine saves millions of lives but, after looking at 30 years of data, the scientists concluded that the DTP vaccine was probably killing more children than died from diphtheria, pertussis and tetanus prior to the vaccine's introduction. The vaccine had ruined the immune systems of children, rendering them susceptible to death from pneumonia, leukaemia, bilharzia, malaria and dysentery. Sadly, the results of that trial changed nothing. The vaccination programmes continued unhindered. The vaccines most often described as having changed the world are those for polio, whooping cough and smallpox. With polio the truth is that as with other infectious diseases the significance of polio dropped as better sanitation, better housing, cleaner water and more food were made available in the second half of the 19th century. Look at the evidence and it shows that the number of polio victims went up not down as a result of vaccination. In Tennessee, USA (chosen at random) the number of polio victims before vaccination became compulsory was 119. The year after vaccination was introduced the figure rose to 386. In America as a whole the number of deaths from polio had fallen dramatically before the first polio vaccine was introduced but the incidence of polio increased by around 50% after the introduction of mass immunisation. Of even more significance, 17 million people who were given polio vaccines as children in the 1950s and 1960s are now at risk of developing cancer. This is because the first practical vaccine used monkey kidney tissue – which contains a carcinogenic virus. Moreover, the virus can be passed on to the children of those who were given the contaminated vaccine. Could this explain the ever rising number of people with cancer? We'll never know. The doctor who first warned of this risk was ignored and her laboratory was closed down. The documents showing who had received the dangerous vaccine were destroyed by the Department of Health in 1987 though it seems likely that millions of doses of the dangerous polio vaccine were used despite the risk. The smallpox story is equally startling. The myth that smallpox was eradicated through a mass vaccination programme is just that – a myth. Smallpox was eradicated through identifying and isolating patients with the disease. One of the worst smallpox epidemics of all time took place in England between 1870 and 1872 – nearly two decades after compulsory vaccination had been introduced. The people of Leicester refused the vaccine and there was only one death. In contrast there were massive numbers of deaths in towns where people had been vaccinated. German doctors are taught that it was the Reich Vaccination Law (making vaccination compulsory) which halted smallpox in their country. But the incidence of smallpox had dropped before the law came into action. Once again, a legally enforced national vaccination programme did not eradicate the disease. Look at history and it is clear that the number of cases of smallpox has gone up each time there has been a mass vaccination programme. It's worth remembering too that Dr Jenner, a hero for pro-vaccine folk, refused to have his second child vaccinated after he'd tried his smallpox vaccination on his own son. Tragically, the boy remained mentally retarded until his death at the age of 21. Everywhere you look the evidence is the same: vaccination doesn't work. Moreover, it is not difficult to sustain the argument that it does more harm than good. Sadly, the medical establishment and the media have for years conspired to suppress the truth and to demonise the truth-tellers – simply demanding bigger and bigger fees for giving vaccinations which have never been properly assessed either for effectiveness or safety.

Thirteenth, the General Medical Council should be closed. A few decades ago the GMC was a modest organisation which existed to weed out doctors who were unworthy. Unfortunately, the disciplinary system was of very little value and concentrated on doctors who had been sleeping with their patients or who had been arrested for offences involving alcohol or drugs. The GMC did very little of value except to provide the newspapers with a good deal of salacious copy. More recently, however, the GMC has, for whatever reason, expanded its interests and its income and has become an industry. The revalidation programme it introduced (arguing that it would exclude incompetent doctors) has done infinitely more harm than good. It is the revalidation programme which has led to many doctors taking early retirement. Closing the GMC would massively improve the quality of health care. It would not be difficult to use police reports to monitor doctors' unacceptable activities and a simple, straightforward complaints system would help exclude those doctors not considered suitable for licensing.

Fourteenth, consultants should be banned from owning (either outright or in shares with other consultants) any private hospital. At the moment, consultants can make massive amounts of money by referring NHS patients to hospitals in which they have shares. It is difficult to see why this is not corrupt.

Fifteenth, drug companies should be banned from sending representatives round to doctors to advertise their products. Doctors who are unable to keep themselves independently educated are not fit to be hired within the NHS. Drug company representatives have traditionally used gifts, meals and holidays to entice doctors to prescribe their products. This is corruption.

Sixteenth, the NHS should revise the system whereby dentists are paid. Some decades ago, dentists were paid far too generously and dentists from other parts of the world (particularly Australia) flooded into the UK to make their fortunes. Since then the pendulum has swung too far the other way. Today, NHS dentistry is second rate and in some parts of the country it is non-existent. It would not be difficult to improve the NHS service so that dentists could make a fair living from working for the NHS.

Seventeenth, nurses working in general practice should go back to working full time in the community. Many now spend much of their time working within surgeries and clinics and doing work which could and should be done by the GP. District nurses should go back to visiting patients at home, providing dressings and treatment and care. The community would benefit enormously from this and many elderly people currently needing to be in sheltered accommodation or care homes would be able to live in their own homes if the district nurse system were revived.

Eighteenth, some of the money saved by firing armies of bureaucrats and dismantling systems which do nothing but further the empire building of administrators could be usefully spent improving the size and quality of the ambulance service. Once GPs are required to go back to providing their patients with a full and decent service, the demand for ambulances would be reduced but there is still room to expand the service. At the moment there are many unemployed doctors in the UK and there is no reason why some of these should not be seconded to work with the ambulance service.

Nineteenth, it has been known for some time that hospitals are dangerous places to be at weekends. The problem is a simple one. The EU's absurd working time regulations mean that young hospital doctors are only allowed to work very limited hours. Indeed, hospitals now employ highly paid administrators to make sure that young doctors only work a certain number of hours. The result is at weekends there are often very few (or even no) doctors working in quite large hospitals. And so no treatment is provided and there are no doctors available to go around the wards to check that all is well.

Twentieth, more time and effort needs to be spent on teaching healthy eating to the public. Simply attempting to ban or discredit certain foods is not enough. The NHS should distribute professionally written information about healthy eating and provide videos on widely visited channels.

Twenty first, hospitals must be stopped from charging patients and visitors to park their cars. Now that small hospitals have been closed (and this is something that should, and could be reversed) patients often have to travel huge distances to attend a hospital. The poor quality of public transport means that patients must drive (or be driven) to hospital in their own motor car. Charging huge car park fees is an unacceptable tax on the sick.

Twenty second, the NHS must stop providing literature and services in several dozen languages. The cost of this is phenomenal. No health care service elsewhere in the world spends money this way. If charities want to provide translators and booklets in other languages that is fine but this is not a responsibility which should be handed over to the NHS.

Twenty third, the NHS must stop providing free treatment for foreigners who come into the UK and demand free treatment. When I was a GP I remember seeing two healthy Germans who came into my surgery and demanded to have operations done free on the NHS. They were in the UK for no more than two weeks and I'm afraid my complex administration procedures (I had to dictate the referral letter and then sign it when it had been typed – usually all on the same day) meant that the Germans had to return home without their free cosmetic surgery. Thousands of people come to the UK to have their babies free of charge or to have operations performed without any cost to themselves. This simply puts up the cost of the NHS and adds to the burden on doctors and hospitals. It also means that UK patients must wait longer for treatment they have paid for.

Twenty fourth, iatrogenic illness needs to be taken seriously. For some years now it has been known that doctors and health care workers are one of the three top causes of death. (The other two are circulatory disorders, such as strokes and heart attacks, and cancer.) Despite this, the damage done by doctors and nurses (largely with drugs and vaccines) is largely ignored. Members of the medical establishment, and their praetorian guard, the experts, always believe they know best. Anyone who questions the establishment must be ignored and, if they persist they must be crushed, suppressed, vilified and ostracised. However, it isn't difficult to compile a litany of medical incompetence – incompetence so egregious that, along with cancer and circulatory disease, doctors have for decades been one of the three most important causes of death and injury. Many of the injuries and deaths among patients are caused by simple, straightforward ignorance and incompetence rather than bad luck or unforeseen complications. The recent enthusiasm for giving millions of patients an untested experimental drug that didn't work and wasn't safe is just one more example of professional ineptitude. If terrorists killed a fraction of the number killed by doctors, the world would be in a state of constant panic. The person most likely to kill you isn't a burglar or an aggrieved relative – it's your doctor. In Australia around half a million people are admitted to hospital every year because they have been made ill by doctors. One in six British hospital patients is in hospital because he or she has been made ill by doctors. Around half of all the 'adverse events' associated with doctors are clearly and readily preventable and are usually a result of ignorance or incompetence or a mixture of both. The rest would be preventable with a little care and thought. Drugs are wildly over-prescribed, both by hospital doctors and by general practitioners. And doctors and hospitals are often appallingly and inexcusably slow. Waiting lists are so long that most patients will now die before they are investigated, let alone treated. Doctors, being human, have always made mistakes but we have now reached the point where, on balance, many apparently well-meaning doctors do more harm than good; killing more people than they are saving and causing more illness and discomfort than they are alleviating. Worryingly, the epidemic of iatrogenic disease which has scarred medical practice for decades has been steadily getting worse. Today most of us would, most of the time, be better off without a medical profession. Major disorders are not picked up in around four out of ten patients. When doctors compared post-mortem results with the patients' medical records they discovered that out of 87 patients, only 17 patients were diagnosed completely correctly. A major study of patients who'd had heart attacks showed that staying at home may be safer than going into hospital. Whatever advantage patients might have had through going into hospital was more than matched by the multiple hazards of being in hospital. Before the industrial age, hospitals were built like cathedrals in order to lift the soul and ease the mind. Hospitals were decorated with works of art, flowers and perfumes. Modern hospitals, designed by experts, are built with no regard for the spirit, eye or soul. They are bare, more like prisons than temples, designed to concentrate the mind on pain, fear and death. In the old days nursing was a noble profession. Caring was the key word. The most powerful jobs in the profession were occupied by ward sisters and matrons — all of whom still had close, daily contact with patients. Today's career structure means that ambitious nurses must move up the ladder to a point where they spend no time with patients. The number of highly paid managers in hospitals has risen every year for decades. There are more administrators in hospitals than there are beds, nurses or other practical staff. A few decades ago patients were cared for in hospitals which were run by matrons and ward sisters — nurses who still knew how to turn a patient, make a bed and empty a bedpan. In many countries, doctors (both in general practice and in hospitals) are now working strictly limited hours. As a result, it is rare to see a doctor in a hospital at weekends. You are up to 26% more likely to die if you are admitted to hospital at the weekend than if you are admitted to hospital during the week. You are more likely to catch a serious, life-threatening infection in hospital than anywhere else. The great danger is, of course, that you may catch an antibiotic resistant infection. Hospitals are poor at hygiene. American researchers have concluded that in an average sort of year surgeons working in American hospitals perform 7.5 million unnecessary surgical procedures, resulting in 37,136 unnecessary deaths and a cost running into hundreds of billions of dollars. One Congressional Committee in the US found that 17.6% of recommendations for surgery were not necessary. Back in 1988, I reported that coronary artery bypass surgery (the commonest procedure performed in cardiac surgery) had been in use for nearly thirty years without anyone trying to find out how patients' everyday lives were affected by the operation. The experts just 'knew' it was a good thing. When a survey was eventually done it was found that the operation had little positive effect on patients' lives but did put a good many patients out of action for some time. And many died as a result of surgical complications. Moreover, patients who have symptoms of heart disease often don't need surgery at all but stand a better chance of recovering if they are put on a regime which includes a vegan diet, gentle exercise and relaxation. Psychiatrists and psychologists are constantly eager to create fashionable new bandwagons and it is now possible to be clinically afraid of over 500 different phobias including korrhaphiophobia (a fear of defeat), apeirophobia (a fear of infinity), chrometophobia (a fear of money) and hippopotomonstrosesquippedaliphobia (a fear of long words). It's difficult to tell when the experts are being serious and when they're having us on. Psychologists have been proved to be worse at making judgements (or offering advice) than hairdressers. Research has shown that psychiatrists are worse than useless. When doctors in Israel went on strike for a month, admissions to hospital dropped by eighty five per cent, with only the most urgent cases being admitted, but despite this the death rate in Israel dropped by fifty per cent — the largest drop since the previous doctors' strike twenty years earlier — to its lowest ever recorded level. Much the same thing happens wherever doctors have gone on strike. The planned and much promoted Great Reset doesn't have a place for doctors or hospitals. An editorial published in the British Medical Journal stated that: 'only one per cent of the articles in medical journals are scientifically sound' and that 'only about fifteen per cent of medical interventions are supported by solid scientific evidence'. Uncomfortable truths (such as those the truth-tellers have been screaming about for the last two years) have always attracted abuse, ridicule and persecution, and those who dare to speak out against the establishment have always been regarded as dangerous heretics. Original thinkers, daring to question the establishment, are still being demonised and cancelled by a modern culture which is just as constrained, as restrictive and as destructive as anything in history. There may not be much burning at the stake going on these days but original thinkers are destroyed by being described as 'conspiracy theorists' or, for absolutely no reason at all, and with no supporting evidence for the slur, labelled as 'discredited'. The licensing authorities remove the licenses of doctors who dare to question the officially approved line of thinking. Doctors who voice views which question drug industry research are told that they must be suffering from mental illness. When I was invited to speak to NHS staff about drug side effects I was banned because the drug industry protested. I was replaced by a drug industry spokesman. I have been banned by YouTube, Facebook, Twitter and the rest of social media, and publishers have banned my books simply because the content was not approved by the establishment. A few years ago, all my books were banned in China after I wrote a column criticising vaccination for a Chinese newspaper. Something similar happened in Germany and several of my books have been banned online because they revealed information which the establishment wanted to keep secret. Still, I mustn't complain. Michael Servetus wrote a book suggesting (accurately) that a separate pulmonary circulation existed within the body. For sharing this truth with the world, Servetus was burnt alive in 1553. These days, doctors just have to put up with censorship and lies and libels online.

Twenty fifth (and although this is last in this list it is certainly not the least important), doctors and hospitals need to start treating the chronically sick, the disabled and the elderly with more respect. On June 18th 2020, I revealed that increasing numbers of patients were being asked to sign Do Not Resuscitate forms or having Do Not Resuscitate forms signed on their behalf. They are known as DNR forms or DNAR forms (for Do Not Attempt Resuscitation). GPs all over the country had been contacting their elderly patients, and those with chronic health disorders, and asking them two questions. 'Are you happy for us to put a DNR on your file?' And: 'Are you happy for us to put on your file a note that you won't be admitted to hospital if you become unwell?' Note the clever wording, designed to elicit a positive response. It's the sort of trickery used by crooked pollsters and insurance salesmen – knowing what answer they want and shading the question in such a way as to ensure that they get it. One GP surgery sent out a letter to a home catering for autistic adults saying that the carers should have plans to prevent their patients being resuscitated if they became critically ill. Other GPs sent out similar letters to establishments caring for the elderly and the disabled. Blanket decisions were made for care homes and residential homes caring for patients with learning difficulties. A 51-year-old man with Down's Syndrome was given a DNR because of his disability, and instructions were left that there was to be no attempt to resuscitate in case of a cardiac arrest or a respiratory arrest. No consent form was signed and there was no agreement with the patient or his relatives. The Medical Director for the relevant part of the NHS said that their policy complied fully with national guidelines from professional bodies. The boss of a large charity said that they believed that DNR orders were frequently being placed on patients with learning disabilities – without the knowledge and agreement of their families. This was, of course, illegal. Back in 2015, the High Court in the UK ruled that carers for patients with mental illnesses should be consulted before DNR notices were applied. But the covid-19 nonsense has resulted in a flood of such cases. A man in his 50s, with sight loss, was issued with a DNR notice giving 'blindness and severe learning disabilities' as the reason. A man with epilepsy was issued with a DNR notice, and a GPs' surgery in Wales urged high risk patients to complete a DNR form if they contracted covid-19. The letter said, 'you are unlikely to receive hospital admission'. A woman in Bristol received a phone call from her GP asking if it were OK for her medical records to be updated to say that if she contracted the covid-19 she wouldn't go to hospital or receive any medical treatment. Is all this really legal? Well, yes, it is if permission is obtained. In the UK, the National Institute for Health and Care Excellence, known as NICE, is the official advisory body to the health care world. And the NICE ruling is utterly crucial. NICE classified people in nine categories. If you are in category 1 then you are very fit. If you are in category 9 then you are terminally ill (though, when it suits them NHS staff sometimes devise another category of 'terminally, terminally ill'). On 29th April 2020, NICE issued amended advice to NHS staff about its resuscitation guidelines, saying that doctors should 'sensitively discuss a possible DNAR with all adults with CFs of 5 or more'. This was issued in response to the coronavirus hoax. Doctors and nurses were instructed that they should review critical care treatment when a patient 'is no longer considered able to achieve desired overall goals'. So, what the devil does this mealy mouthed nonsense mean? And what is a CF? What does a CF of 5 mean? Well the letters CF mean clinical frailty and there are several stages. A CF of 5 means that a patient is mildly frail and may need help with heavy housework, shopping and preparing meals. A CF of 6 means moderately frail – people who need help with bathing. A CF of 7 means severely frail – people who are completely dependent for personal care. And so on. Now you could, I suppose, argue that if a patient is clearly dying then it would be cruel and pointless to continually attempt resuscitation. That was why DNR notices were devised. They were originally for patients who had only hours to live and it was considered not fair to those patients to continue to 'strive to keep officiously alive'. But that's not what is happening now. Today, in the UK, in the National Health Service, a patient who needs help with the heavy housework and who may have difficulty preparing meals or going to the shops is not considered worth treating. I could manage a bit of light dusting, I suppose, but more than that would require more effort than I have available. I would have great difficulty in preparing a meal and I hate going to the shops. So, presumably, I'd get dumped into the CF5 category and so there is no hope for me, and the NHS would recommend that I be denied antibiotics, painkillers or surgery if I fell down and broke an arm. Today, the NHS doesn't want to save anyone who is disabled and all patients in care homes are, by definition, suitable for murder by omission. Originally NICE told doctors that they should assess patients with autism as scoring high for frailty. I am, I confess, still rather confused about when or whether this advice was removed. I checked around with other bodies. I didn't find the BMA website much help, though it did have a useful commercial webinar for doctors wanting financial advice. The BMA is, after all, a trades union which exists to look after doctors not patients. And the General Medical Council, rather bizarrely, got in on the act by defining 'approaching end of life' as patients who are likely to die within the next twelve months. This, of course is the sort of dangerous rubbish one might expect from the overpaid bureaucratic form shufflers at the General Medical Council because it is always impossible to say that a patient is likely to die within twelve months. It may be possible to say that a patient might die within twelve hours but not twelve months. Only arrogant doctors and ignorant bureaucrats claim to know that a patient might die within twelve months. When I was in general practice, I knew many patients who were given months to live but who lived many, many years. Two, I remember well, had young children to look after and although they had been given only months to live they both lived for years – simply refusing to give up and surviving on sheer willpower as much as anything else. If the GMC rule had been applied, they'd have been allowed to die. Or, the way things seem to be going, they would have been quietly euthanized in case they fell ill and needed care. While digging around I also found this statement: 'Physicians have been empowered to grant a mercy death to patients considered incurable – the mentally ill and the handicapped.' And then I looked a little closer and realised that the date of that policy statement was October 1939, and the author was a well-known 'medical expert' known as Adolf Hitler. Hitler's policy, which seems to me to bear an uncomfortably close relationship to the official policy of the UK's National Health Service these days, was created in 1920 in a book written by a psychiatrist and a lawyer (what a deadly combination) who argued that the economic savings justified killing those with 'useless lives'. The policy was to kill the incurably ill and the physically or mentally disabled and the elderly. Hitler's policy was officially discontinued in 1941 when it seems that even the Nazis found it a bit much. But the advice from NICE is still valid. And the NHS is still prepared to refuse life-saving treatment for the elderly, the disabled or the frail. Refusing treatment to patients solely because of their age or fitness is a form of eugenics. It seems that social cleansing is alive and well in Britain today. If you aren't saving people (when you could do so) then you are killing them. There doesn't seem to me to be all that much difference between the thinking behind the policy of the NHS and the policy of Adolf Hitler's Germany. If you slap a DNR form on a patient, with or without their permission, you are condemning them to death. If you trick someone into agreeing to one then that's just as bad. In my view, the NHS has been Nazified. There are many good doctors and nurses working for it. But there are many who are so bad they are evil. Which of us gave doctors permission to behave like Nazis and to deny treatment to people considered unimportant, expensive or expendable? In my view, every single doctor or nurse or administrator who has put a DNR notice on a patient under these regulations should be fired, arrested and imprisoned. I am prepared to believe that not everyone in health care can have a genuine vocation. But the 'experts' who are scattering these DNR notices around are paid to look after people. And they have betrayed those people. Do Not Resuscitate notices were devised to ensure that the genuinely terminally ill were allowed to die with dignity – without being dragged time and time again from wherever they were heading. DNR notices were originally a necessary part of medicine – to avoid General Franco type situations. But now we have a thousand Dr Mengele clones working in the health service and millions of elderly citizens are terrified of falling ill and needing to go into hospital because they know that if they go in then there is a very good chance that they will never come out. That sounds as if I'm exaggerating but the sad thing is that I am not. Dr Mengele would have thrived in today's NHS. He'd have liked the clapping and the adulation too. NICE should be disbanded immediately. We'd all be better off without it. Meanwhile, if you think you, or someone you know could be rated C5 or worse, it might be a good idea to ask your GP if you've been put on the 'suitable for dying' list.

There are more things that could and should be done. But that's just a start. If all these changes were made then the NHS would be revived and transformed.

Sadly, of course, you and I both know none of these things will happen because there are just too many vested interest groups controlling the NHS. Politicians are scared of doing anything other than praise the NHS because they believe it is popular with the electorate. Doctors don't want to change anything because they are under-worked and overpaid. The same is due of nurses. The trade unions representing doctors, nurses and other professionals will fight tooth and nail to maintain the status quo – however damaging it is for patients. Drug companies constantly cheat the NHS out of millions of pounds by overcharging and have been doing this for decades. Occasionally, a big drug company will be charged a few million pounds for over-charging. This doesn't seem to change things. The fines seem to be regarded as nothing more than an annoying cost of doing business.

But there is a viable and valid alternative: a health care system which could replace the NHS and provide everyone in the country with much better health care – without costing a penny more.

# Part Three
## A Better Alternative

The only way to do something about the health care crisis is to provide the public with enough information so that they demand that politicians act. It is only politicians (given support from the public) who can possibly ever replace an organisation which is basically corrupt and dangerous and which has failed its customers (the patients).

The key figures which need to be widely shared are these:

First, the amount of money which taxpayers spend on the NHS is, for 2021-22, £193 billion (this figure does not include benefit payments of various kinds).

Second, the number of people living in the UK is currently 67,886,004.

A moment with a calculator shows that taxpayers in the UK are paying the NHS £2,838 a head for looking after each man, woman and child in the country. That covers the third rate service offered by general practitioners and the second rate service offered by hospitals.

And this is where it becomes interesting because with just under £3,000 a head available to spend on health care, every individual and every family in the country could buy themselves excellent, comprehensive private health cover – cover that would entitle them to the services of a GP, available 24 hours a day and 365 days a year, and to treatment in a private hospital of their choice if needed.

How can this possibly be?

Simple.

The NHS is the most bureaucratic, over-staffed organisation in the world. Remove the many thousands of unnecessary (and very expensive) administrators and the costs plummet.

Here's how it would work.

First, the Government would allocate £2,838 in health vouchers (like luncheon vouchers if you will) to every individual in the country. A family of four would receive four times that sum, and so on. The full £2,838 would be available for every man, woman and child – regardless of sex or age.

Those doctors wanting to work as general practitioners (or, as I prefer it, family doctors) would simply set up in their own locality and offer their services to patients. All family doctors in an area would, of course, be in competition with one another to provide the best service. There would be no need for any central administration.

And so, for example, Dr Brownlow (a name taken from my books about the village of Bilbury in North Devon) might say to his potential patients that he would make himself available for consultations, home visits and telephone calls for 24 hours a day, 365 days a year. He would announce that he was working in partnership with two other local doctors and that if he was not available (because he was having the evening off, or taking a holiday) then one of his partners would be available in his absence. There would always be a doctor available for a consultation or a home visit and the patient would choose whether he or she wanted to be seen at home or in the surgery. (This would save Dr Brownlow a good deal of money because he wouldn't need a big clinic or a great many members of staff. He could turn a room in his home into a consulting room and hire his wife to answer the phone in his absence – just as used to happen in the early days of the NHS. These days, of course, she could hire her husband to do these things.)

'How much will this cost me?' will be the first question a potential patient might ask.

'I would expect you to pay me by direct debit,' Dr Brownlow might reply. 'And I'd like a monthly payment of £20 per person. That's £240 a year. For that I will provide all the medical services you require from me and you will receive all basic medicines – such as antibiotics and painkillers – at no extra charge. If you need very unusual and expensive medicines that will be covered by a small insurance policy costing just £10 a year. If you need an operation or specialist advice then I will arrange for you to be seen by a consultant specialist at one of the local private hospitals. This will be paid for through your hospital insurance scheme.'

'So I will have to pay you even when I am well?' the prospective patient will ask.

'Yes,' Dr Brownlow will reply. 'That is the way that doctors always used to be paid in sophisticated cultures. And it's the way the NHS used to operate. You paid your taxes whether you were ill or well.'

'How many patients will you be looking after?' will be an obvious question from the prospective patient.

'I will have no more than 500 patients,' Dr Brownlow will reply. 'My practice will close when I have 500 patients. That will give me an income of £120,000 a year which will be, after my modest expenses, around the same as I earn at the moment from the NHS. You will benefit because with just 500 patients to look after I will know you and your family and I will have far more time to spend with you. And I will benefit because although I will be available at all times I will have a much smaller list of patients to care for, I will be able to enjoy the work I was trained for and I will have virtually no boring and time consuming paperwork to complete. There will, of course, be no complicated appointments system to manage and I, or one of my two partners, will see every patient either immediately or within hours of their wanting to see me.'

'But what if I need to go to hospital for an operation or treatment?' the patient will ask.

'Your hospital cover will be provided by BUPA or PPP or one of the other big health insurance companies,' Dr Brownlow will reply. 'They will all be required by law to offer hospital cover at the same price whatever your personal medical history or age might be. After paying me £250 a year (including the £10 for rare drugs insurance cover) you will have £2,588 a year for hospital cover. You will find that you will be able to buy excellent cover with that amount of money available. A family of four will have £10,352 available. If you like I can arrange the cover for you to make sure that you have the best local hospitals and specialists available. The bill for hospital cover will be much lower than the sum available and so there will be vouchers available for use if you want to access alternative or complementary medical services.'

And it will be as simple as that.

Everyone will benefit. It's a win-win situation for every patient and every doctor.

The only losers will be the administrators who currently suck up most of the money allocated to the NHS.

They will have to find useful jobs outside the health sector.

## Books by Vernon Coleman include:

### Medical
The Medicine Men
Paper Doctors
Everything You Want To Know About Ageing
The Home Pharmacy
Aspirin or Ambulance
Face Values
Stress and Your Stomach
A Guide to Child Health
Guilt
The Good Medicine Guide
An A to Z of Women's Problems
Bodypower
Bodysense
Taking Care of Your Skin
Life without Tranquillisers
High Blood Pressure
Diabetes
Arthritis
Eczema and Dermatitis
The Story of Medicine
Natural Pain Control
Mindpower
Addicts and Addictions
Dr Vernon Coleman's Guide to Alternative Medicine
Stress Management Techniques
Overcoming Stress
The Health Scandal
The 20 Minute Health Check
Sex for Everyone
Mind over Body
Eat Green Lose Weight
Why Doctors Do More Harm Than Good
The Drugs Myth

Complete Guide to Sex
How to Conquer Backache
How to Conquer Pain
Betrayal of Trust
Know Your Drugs
Food for Thought
The Traditional Home Doctor
Relief from IBS
The Parent's Handbook
Men in Bras, Panties and Dresses
Power over Cancer
How to Conquer Arthritis
How to Stop Your Doctor Killing You
Superbody
Stomach Problems – Relief at Last
How to Overcome Guilt
How to Live Longer
Coleman's Laws
Millions of Alzheimer Patients Have Been Misdiagnosed
Climbing Trees at 112
Is Your Health Written in the Stars?
The Kick-Ass A–Z for over 60s
Briefs Encounter
The Benzos Story
Dementia Myth
Medical Heretics

## Psychology/Sociology
Stress Control
How to Overcome Toxic Stress
Know Yourself (1988)
Stress and Relaxation
People Watching
Spiritpower
Toxic Stress
I Hope Your Penis Shrivels Up
Oral Sex: Bad Taste and Hard To Swallow
Other People's Problems

The 100 Sexiest, Craziest, Most Outrageous Agony Column Questions (and Answers) Of All Time
How to Relax and Overcome Stress
Too Sexy To Print
Psychiatry
Are You Living With a Psychopath?

## Politics and General
England Our England
Rogue Nation
Confronting the Global Bully
Saving England
Why Everything Is Going To Get Worse Before It Gets Better
The Truth They Won't Tell You...About The EU
Living In a Fascist Country
How to Protect & Preserve Your Freedom, Identity & Privacy
Oil Apocalypse
Gordon is a Moron
The OFPIS File
What Happens Next?
Bloodless Revolution
2020
Stuffed
The Shocking History of the EU
Coming Apocalypse
Covid-19: The Greatest Hoax in History
Old Man in a Chair
Endgame
Proof that Masks do more harm than Good
Covid-19: The Fraud Continues
Covid-19: Exposing the Lies
Social Credit: Nightmare on Your Street
NHS: What's wrong and how to put it right
Diaries and Autobiographies
Diary of a Disgruntled Man
Just another Bloody Year
Bugger off and Leave Me Alone
Return of the Disgruntled Man

Life on the Edge
The Game's Afoot
Tickety Tonk
Memories 1
Memories 2

## Animals
Why Animal Experiments Must Stop
Fighting For Animals
Alice and Other Friends
Animal Rights – Human Wrongs
Animal Experiments – Simple Truths

## General Non Fiction
How to Publish Your Own Book
How to Make Money While Watching TV
Strange but True
Daily Inspirations
Why Is Public Hair Curly
People Push Bottles Up Peaceniks
Secrets of Paris
Moneypower
101 Things I Have Learned
100 Greatest Englishmen and Englishwomen
Cheese Rolling, Shin Kicking and Ugly Tattoos
One Thing after Another
My Favourite Books

## Novels (General)
Mrs Caldicot's Cabbage War
Mrs Caldicot's Knickerbocker Glory
Mrs Caldicot's Oyster Parade
Mrs Caldicot's Turkish Delight
Deadline
Second Chance
Tunnel
Mr Henry Mulligan
The Truth Kills

Revolt
My Secret Years with Elvis
Balancing the Books
Doctor in Paris
Stories with a Twist in the Tale (short stories)
Dr Bullock's Annals

## The Young Country Doctor Series
Bilbury Chronicles
Bilbury Grange
Bilbury Revels
Bilbury Country
Bilbury Village
Bilbury Pie (short stories)
Bilbury Pudding (short stories)
Bilbury Tonic
Bilbury Relish
Bilbury Mixture
Bilbury Delights
Bilbury Joys
Bilbury Tales
Bilbury Days
Bilbury Memories

## Novels (Sport)
Thomas Winsden's Cricketing Almanack
Diary of a Cricket Lover
The Village Cricket Tour
The Man Who Inherited a Golf Course
Around the Wicket
Too Many Clubs and Not Enough Balls

## Cat books
Alice's Diary
Alice's Adventures
We Love Cats
Cats Own Annual
The Secret Lives of Cats

Cat Basket
The Cataholics' Handbook
Cat Fables
Cat Tales
Catoons from Catland

## As Edward Vernon
Practice Makes Perfect
Practise What You Preach
Getting Into Practice
Aphrodisiacs – An Owner's Manual
The Complete Guide to Life

## Written with Donna Antoinette Coleman
How to Conquer Health Problems between Ages 50 & 120
Health Secrets Doctors Share With Their Families
Animal Miscellany
England's Glory
Wisdom of Animals

## Note from the Author:

If you found this book informative I would be very grateful if you would put a suitable review online. It helps more than you can imagine. If you disliked the book, or disapproved of it in any way, please forget you read it.
Vernon Coleman

Printed in Great Britain
by Amazon